Pelvic Floor Exercises for Senior Women

The Illustrated Guides to Easy Kegel Exercises to Heal Incontinence, Pain, and Prolapse

OLIVIA HOYLES

Disclaimer

The recipes in this book are for informational purposes only. While every effort has been made to ensure accuracy, the author takes no responsibility for any injuries or illnesses arising from the use of the information provided.

TABLE OF CONTENTS

Introduction

Taking Charge of Your Wellbeing with Pelvic Floor Exercises

Imagine yourself at your favorite park, enjoying a brisk walk with friends. Suddenly, you feel a familiar **tightness** – **a sneeze** you weren't expecting might lead to **a leak.** Or, perhaps you struggle with holding back the urge to use the restroom, making outings a bit stressful.

These are common experiences for many senior women, often attributed to **"just getting older."** But what if there was a way to regain control and rediscover confidence?

The answer lies in a group of muscles you might not even realize exist – your pelvic floor muscles. Think of them as a hidden hammock, cradling your bladder, uterus, and rectum. Strong pelvic floor muscles provide vital support for these organs, **promoting bladder** and **bowel control**, **sexual health**, and **even core stability.**

Meet Mary, an Active Senior:

Mary, a vibrant 72-year-old, loved her weekly Zumba classes. But lately, the fear of leaks kept her on the sidelines. Pelvic floor exercises became her secret weapon. Within a few weeks, she noticed a significant improvement in her bladder control, allowing her to confidently return to her Zumba class and reconnect with her friends.

Why Are Pelvic Floor Muscles Important? The Hidden Hammock Supporting Your Wellbeing

Imagine a hidden hammock cradling your bladder, uterus, and rectum. That's essentially what your pelvic floor muscles are – a network of muscles that provide vital support and stability for your entire pelvic region. Strong pelvic floor muscles play a crucial role in many aspects of your health, and understanding their importance is key to maintaining well-being throughout life, especially as we age.

The Symphony of Support:

Think of your pelvic floor like an orchestra conductor, coordinating the smooth operation of several vital functions:

Bladder Control: Strong pelvic floor muscles help you control the flow of urine. They act like a sphincter, tightening around the urethra (the tube that carries urine from the bladder) to prevent leaks during activities that put pressure on your abdomen, like coughing, sneezing, or laughing.

❖ **Bowel Control:** Similarly, your pelvic floor muscles work with the anal sphincter to control the passage of stool, preventing accidental bowel movements.

❖ **Pelvic Organ Support:** These muscles act as a hammock, supporting the weight of your bladder, uterus, and rectum. Weak pelvic floor muscles can lead to a condition called pelvic organ prolapse, where these organs may bulge or descend into the vagina.

❖ **Sexual Function:** Pelvic floor muscles play a significant role in sexual health for both men and women. Strong pelvic floor muscles can enhance sexual arousal, pleasure, and orgasm intensity.

❖ **Core Stability:** Your pelvic floor works in conjunction with your core muscles to provide overall stability and support for your spine. Weak pelvic floor muscles can contribute to back pain and poor posture.

The Effects of Weakening:

Your pelvic floor muscles may become weaker for a number of reasons, such as:

❖ **Pregnancy and childbirth:** The weight of the baby and the stress of childbirth can stretch and weaken the pelvic floor muscles.

❖ **Menopause:** Decreased estrogen levels can contribute to weakened pelvic floor muscles.

❖ **Chronic straining:** Constipation, heavy lifting, or chronic coughing can put excess strain on your pelvic floor muscles, leading to weakness.

❖ **Surgery:** Pelvic surgeries can sometimes damage or weaken the pelvic floor muscles.

When Weakness Becomes a Concern:

Weakness in your pelvic floor muscles can manifest in several ways:

❖ **Urinary incontinence:** Leaking pee while exercising, sneezing, or coughing.

❖ **Pelvic organ prolapses:** A feeling of heaviness or pressure in the vagina, or a bulge protruding from the vagina.

❖ **Bowel incontinence:** Difficulty controlling stool.

❖ Sexual dysfunction: Decreased sensation, pain during intercourse, or difficulty achieving orgasm.

❖ **Back pain:** Weakness in the pelvic floor can contribute to back pain and poor posture.

The best part is that you don't have to wait until you experience these issues to take action. Pelvic floor exercises, also known as Kegels, can strengthen these muscles and prevent problems in the future. Even if you're already experiencing some weakness, it's never too late to see improvement!

Chapter 2: Benefits of Pelvic Floor Exercises for Senior Women

The good news? It's never too late to strengthen your pelvic floor muscles and reclaim control of your wellbeing.

As women age, our bodies go through incredible changes. While some changes are inevitable, weak pelvic floor muscles don't have to be one of them. Pelvic floor exercises, often referred to as Kegels, offer a powerful and natural way to strengthen these muscles, leading to a range of benefits that can significantly improve your quality of life.

Let's explore in more detail how these easy activities might open up a world of wellbeing for older women:

1. Regaining Bladder and Bowel Control:

One of the most life-altering benefits of strong pelvic floor muscles is improved bladder and bowel control. Many women experience stress incontinence, a sudden leak of urine during activities like coughing, laughing, or exercise. This can be incredibly frustrating and lead to social isolation. Strengthening your pelvic floor muscles helps you regain control of your bladder, allowing you to participate fully in activities you enjoy without fear of leaks.

Meet Agnes, a Social Butterfly:

Agnes, a vivacious 68-year-old, loved attending social gatherings. However, the constant worry about leaks kept her on the edge of her seat. Pelvic floor exercises became **her secret weapon.** Within a few months, she noticed a significant improvement in her bladder control, allowing her to confidently rejoin social circles and reconnect with friends. She now enjoys attending events without the constant worry of leaks.

2. Enhanced Sexual Function:

The muscles of the pelvic floor are essential for healthy sexual behavior. Robust pelvic floor muscles may result in:

→ **Increased sensation:** Improved blood flow to the genital area can heighten sexual arousal and pleasure.

→ **Stronger orgasms:** Contractions of the pelvic floor muscles during orgasm can be more intense and satisfying.

→ **Better lubrication:** Stronger pelvic floor muscles can improve vaginal lubrication, making sex more comfortable.

3. Reduced Back Pain:

The pelvic floor muscles work in conjunction with your core muscles to provide overall stability and support for your spine. Weak pelvic floor muscles can contribute to back pain. By strengthening your pelvic floor, you can improve your core stability, potentially reducing back pain and improving your posture.

4. Increased Overall Well-being:

The benefits of pelvic floor exercises extend far beyond physical improvements. Regaining control of your bladder and bowel function, experiencing a more fulfilling sex life, and reducing back pain can all contribute to a significant improvement in your overall well-being. You'll feel more empowered, confident, and in control of your body, allowing you to embrace life to the fullest.

5. A Preventive Measure:

Pelvic floor exercises are not just about addressing existing issues; they're also a fantastic preventative measure. By strengthening your pelvic floor muscles proactively, you can reduce your risk of developing problems like incontinence and prolapse later in life.

Addressing Common Concerns:

Taking charge of your pelvic floor health is an empowering step. But it's normal to have doubts and worries. Let's address some of the most common anxieties senior women face when considering pelvic floor exercises:

1. "I Won't Be Able to Feel the Muscles"

This is a frequent worry, and it's completely understandable! The pelvic floor muscles are internal, making them a little trickier to locate compared to a bicep. These pointers can assist you in recognizing them:

Imagine stopping your urine flow midstream (don't actually do this!): The muscles you use to do this are your pelvic floor muscles.

The "squeeze and lift" test: While lying down, gently squeeze your vagina as if you're trying to hold back urine or gas. There ought to be a mild lifting feeling.

If you're still unsure, don't hesitate to consult a healthcare professional. They can help you identify the correct muscles and ensure you're performing the exercises effectively.

2. "These Exercises Won't Work for Me at My Age"

This is a myth! Your body is incredibly responsive, and consistent exercise, regardless of age, can lead to significant improvements. Studies have shown that even women who begin pelvic floor exercises later in life experience positive results, including improved bladder control and increased sexual satisfaction.

3. "Pelvic Floor Exercises Sound Too Clinical"

They don't have to be! The beauty of these exercises is their simplicity and discretion. They may be done discreetly and anyplace, at any time. Here are some ways to integrate them into your daily routine:

While watching TV: Squeeze and hold your pelvic floor muscles during commercial breaks.

Waiting in line: Do a few quick pelvic floor contractions while you wait your turn.

During your commute: Discreetly contract your pelvic floor muscles while sitting on the bus or train.

4. "I'm Embarrassed to Talk About This"

Remember, you're not alone! Pelvic floor issues are incredibly common among senior women. Medical personnel are there to assist you, not to pass judgment. Talking openly about your concerns can lead to effective treatment and improved quality of life.

5. "I Don't Know Where to Start"

This guide is a great starting point! We'll provide detailed instructions on performing pelvic floor exercises correctly. There are also many online resources and instructional videos available. Consider consulting a physical therapist specializing in pelvic floor health – they can create a personalized exercise routine tailored to your specific needs.

Note

It's a marathon, not a sprint. Consistency is key to seeing results. Start slowly and gradually increase the duration and intensity of your exercises as you get stronger.

Be patient with yourself. It may take a few weeks or even months to notice a significant difference.

This guide will equip you with the knowledge and confidence to embark on a journey of strengthening your pelvic floor muscles.

Chapter 3: Locating Your Pelvic Floor Muscles

The Key to Effective Exercises

Before embarking on your pelvic floor exercise journey, it's crucial to identify the muscles you'll be targeting. While they may feel like a hidden mystery at first, there are a couple of techniques you can use to locate them, both with and without a trip to the bathroom.

The Restroom Technique:

This method utilizes the natural function of urination to help you identify the pelvic floor muscles. However, it's important to avoid actually interrupting your urine flow, as this can disrupt your natural rhythm and potentially lead to urinary tract infections.

1. **Settle in:** Sit comfortably on the toilet as if you're about to urinate.
2. **Imagine stopping the flow:** Without actually stopping your urine stream, try to imagine you're clenching the muscles that

would allow you to do so midstream. You should feel a tightening sensation in your pelvic floor.

3. **Focus on the feeling:** Hold this contraction for a few seconds, then relax. Focus on the internal movement and identify the muscles involved.

The Non-Restroom Technique:

This method allows you to locate your pelvic floor muscles without using the restroom. It may take a bit more practice, but it's a convenient way to become familiar with these internal muscles.

1. **Get comfortable:** Lie down on your back with your knees bent and feet flat on the floor. Alternatively, you can sit upright in a chair.

2. **Imagine a lift:** Imagine you're trying to lift your pelvic floor up towards your navel. You should feel a subtle tightening sensation in the vagina and rectum area.

3. **Squeeze and hold:** Once you've identified the sensation, gently squeeze these

muscles as if you're trying to hold back gas. Hold for a few seconds, then relax.

1. Get comfortable
2. Imagine a lift
3. Squeeze and hold

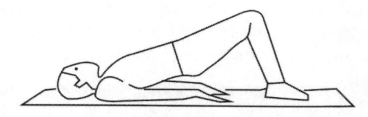

The Non-Restroom Technique

Additional Tips:

Don't confuse it with clenching: Avoid clenching your buttocks or abdominal muscles. The focus should be solely on the internal pelvic floor muscles.

Imagine a cough hold: Another way to think about it is to imagine you're holding back a cough. The muscles you use for that are your pelvic floor muscles.

Practice makes perfect: Don't get discouraged if you don't feel anything immediately. It may take some practice to isolate the correct muscles.

Beyond Feeling:

While feeling the pelvic floor muscles is ideal, it's not essential for everyone. Some women may have difficulty feeling them initially. Here are ways to confirm you're on the right track:

Observe external changes: During the contraction, you may notice a slight inward movement of the lower abdomen or buttocks.

Use a biofeedback device: These devices can provide visual or auditory feedback to confirm if you're contracting the correct muscles. These can be helpful for beginners but are not always necessary.

The key is to focus on the internal sensation of tightening and lifting. With a little patience and practice, you'll be able to locate your pelvic floor muscles.

Proper Breathing and Posture

The Powerful Link: Why Proper Breathing and Posture Matter for Pelvic Floor Health

When it comes to strengthening your pelvic floor muscles and optimizing your overall well-being, two often-overlooked factors play a crucial role: proper breathing and posture. They may seem unrelated, but they're intricately connected to the health of your pelvic floor. Here's why:

The Breath of Life:

Enhanced Oxygen Flow: Deep, diaphragmatic breathing (breathing from your belly) allows your diaphragm, a dome-shaped muscle below your lungs, to move efficiently. This optimizes oxygen intake, which is vital for all your muscles, including your pelvic floor.

Improved Blood Flow: Deep breathing promotes better circulation throughout your body, delivering essential nutrients and oxygen to your pelvic floor muscles, keeping them healthy and strong.

Reduced Stress Response: Chronic shallow breathing is often linked to stress, which can lead to muscle tension, including in the pelvic floor. Deep breathing promotes relaxation, allowing your pelvic floor muscles to function optimally.

The Power of Posture:

Optimal Alignment: Good posture means your body is positioned in a way that minimizes stress on your muscles and joints. This includes maintaining a neutral spine and avoiding slouching or hunching. When your posture is right, your pelvic floor muscles are naturally supported, allowing them to function more effectively.

Improved Core Engagement: Good posture activates your core muscles, which work in conjunction with your pelvic floor muscles to provide stability and support for your entire torso and pelvis. Engaging your core during exercises can also enhance the effectiveness of pelvic floor exercises.

Reduced Strain: Poor posture, especially slouching or arching your back, can put undue strain on your pelvic floor muscles. This can lead to weakness, discomfort, and even contribute to issues like incontinence.

The Synergy:

Think of proper breathing and posture as the foundation for a strong pelvic floor.

Deep breathing provides the necessary oxygen and relaxation for your pelvic floor muscles to function effectively.

Good posture ensures optimal alignment and reduces strain on these muscles, making them more responsive to exercises.

Benefits Beyond the Pelvic Floor:

The positive effects of proper breathing and posture extend far beyond your pelvic floor health:

Improved Overall Fitness: Deep breathing increases oxygen intake, which can enhance your athletic performance and endurance.

Reduced Back Pain: Good posture helps maintain proper spinal alignment, leading to less back pain and improved flexibility.

Enhanced Energy Levels: Deep breathing and good posture promote better circulation, which can leave you feeling more energized throughout the day.

Stress Reduction: Focusing on deep breathing techniques can help calm your mind and reduce stress levels.

Tips for Success:

Practice Deep Breathing: Focus on breathing from your belly, not your chest. Imagine your belly inflating like a balloon with each inhale, and gently deflate with each exhale.

Mind Your Posture: Stand tall with your shoulders back and relaxed, your core engaged, and your weight evenly distributed on both feet.

Incorporate Both: While performing pelvic floor exercises, focus on maintaining good posture and incorporate deep breathing techniques. Inhale before contracting your pelvic floor muscles, and exhale as you relax.

Chapter 4: Choosing Comfortable Positions for Exercises

The Key to Pelvic Floor Success

Pelvic floor exercises, also known as Kegels, can be done anywhere, anytime. However, choosing comfortable positions is crucial for proper technique and maximizing the effectiveness of your workout. Here's a guide to help you find the perfect positions for optimal results:

The Power of Comfort:

Mind-Muscle Connection: When you're comfortable, you can focus on isolating and contracting the correct muscles – your pelvic floor. Discomfort can distract you and make it harder to perform the exercises correctly.

Strong pelvic floor exercises require relaxed surrounding muscles. If you're tense or uncomfortable, it can be difficult to fully engage and relax your pelvic floor muscles.

Comfort plays a key role in consistency. If certain positions are uncomfortable, you're less likely to stick with your exercise routine. Finding comfortable positions makes it easier to integrate pelvic floor exercises seamlessly into your daily life.

Exploring Your Options:

Here are some excellent positions to consider for your pelvic floor exercises:

Lying Down: This is a classic and comfortable position for beginners. Lie on your back with your knees bent and feet flat on the floor. This position helps isolate your pelvic floor muscles and minimize strain.

Sitting in a Chair: Sitting upright in a chair with good posture can also be a comfortable option. Ensure your back is straight and your feet are flat on the floor. This is a discreet position allowing you to exercise throughout the day.

Standing Tall: Once you're comfortable with the exercises, standing tall with good posture can be another option. This position engages your core muscles and allows you to practice pelvic floor activation in a functional way.

Finding What Works for You:

Try different positions and see what feels most comfortable for you. There's no "one size fits all" approach, so experiment until you find a sweet spot. Stop doing the workout right away if you feel any pain or discomfort. Adjust your position or try a different exercise altogether.

As you get stronger, you can gradually progress to more challenging positions. Don't force yourself into uncomfortable positions – focus on maintaining good form and technique.

Making it Enjoyable:

Create a Routine: Choose a time of day that works for you and incorporate pelvic floor exercises into your daily routine.

Multitasking Magic: Integrate Kegels into your daily activities. Do them while watching TV, waiting in line, or even while standing at work.

Mindfulness Matters: Focus on the sensation of your pelvic floor muscles contracting and relaxing. This mindfulness can make the exercises more engaging and help you track your progress.

The goal is to find comfortable positions that allow you to isolate and strengthen your pelvic floor muscles effectively.

Chapter 5: Core Exercises

Kegel Exercises: The Cornerstone of Pelvic Floor Strength

Kegel exercises, named after Dr. Arnold Kegel, are the foundation of a strong pelvic floor. These simple yet powerful exercises involve contracting and relaxing the muscles that support your bladder, uterus, and rectum. While they may seem straightforward, proper technique is key to maximizing their effectiveness. Let's delve deeper into the world of Kegels and guide you towards optimal pelvic floor health:

Understanding the Muscles:

Before diving into the exercises, it's helpful to understand the target muscles. Imagine a hammock cradling your pelvic organs – that's essentially what your pelvic floor muscles do. **These muscles include:**

Levator Ani: This is the main group of muscles targeted during Kegels. They form a sling-like structure supporting your pelvic organs.

Sphincter Muscles: These muscles surround the urethra (urine passage) and anus, helping control urination and bowel movements.

The Power of Kegels:

Here's how to do Kegel exercises correctly, step-by-step:

1. **Locate the Muscles**: As discussed earlier, use the restroom technique or the non-restroom technique to identify your pelvic floor muscles.

2. **Get Comfortable:** Choose a comfortable position, either lying down, sitting, or standing. Remember, good posture is essential.

3. **The Squeeze:** Imagine you're trying to stop your urine flow midstream (without actually doing so). Gently squeeze your pelvic floor muscles upwards and inwards. Hold this contraction for a count of 2-3 seconds.

4. **Relax and Repeat:** Relax your pelvic floor muscles completely. Repeat the squeeze and hold for 2-3 seconds, aiming for 10 repetitions per set.

5. **Focus on Quality, not Quantity**: It's more important to focus on contracting the correct muscles with proper form than doing a large number of repetitions with poor technique.

6. **Breathe Easy:** Continue breathing normally throughout the exercise. Don't hold your breath while contracting your muscles.

Repeat the squeeze and hold for:

2-3 seconds

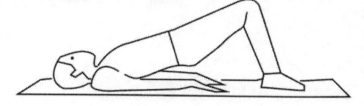

Aim for 10 repetitions per set.

Building a Routine:

Here are some tips for incorporating Kegel exercises seamlessly into your daily life:

→ Begin with 3 sets of 10 repetitions daily. Gradually increase the duration of holds (up to 10 seconds) and the number of repetitions per set (up to 15) as you get stronger.

→ Aim to perform your Kegels daily, even if it's just a few sets. Consistency is crucial for seeing results.

→ Integrate Kegels into your daily routine. Do them while brushing your teeth, waiting in line, or watching TV.

If you experience any pain or discomfort, stop immediately and consult your healthcare professional.

Variations for Added Challenge:

Once you've mastered the basic Kegel exercise, consider these variations to further challenge your pelvic floor muscles:

Short Pulses: Instead of holding the contraction, perform quick squeezes and relaxes of your pelvic floor muscles.

Quick Flicks: Contract your pelvic floor muscles very quickly and then relax completely. Repeat this several times.

Pulsing Holds: During the hold, perform small, pulsing contractions within the main squeeze.

Chapter 6: Pilates exercises for pelvic floor

PELVIC TILTS:

1. **Starting Position:** Lie on your back, bend your knees and place your feet flat on the ground while lying on your back. Your hands need to be at your sides, facing downward.

2. **Inhale to Prepare:** Take a deep breath in, allowing your abdomen to expand and your lower back to gently arch away from the floor.

3. **Exhale and Engage:** As you exhale, tilt your pelvis upward by pressing your lower back into the floor. Imagine pulling your pubic bone towards your belly button, engaging your pelvic floor muscles.

4. **Hold and Release:** Hold the contraction for a few seconds, feeling the engagement in your pelvic floor. Then, inhale to release back to the neutral starting position.

5. **Repeat:** Perform 10-15 repetitions, focusing on smooth and controlled movements with each tilt.

Hold: Few Seconds

Repeat: 10-15 rep

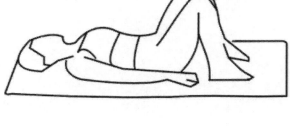

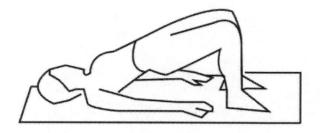

PELVIC TILTS

Why You'll Feel the Difference:

Pelvic tilts help to strengthen and stabilize the muscles of the pelvic floor, lower back, and abdomen. They also promote better posture by encouraging awareness of pelvic alignment. Engaging the pelvic floor during the tilt, you improve muscle tone and support for the pelvic organs, which can help alleviate symptoms of pelvic floor dysfunction such as urinary incontinence or pelvic pain.

BRIDGE:

1. **Starting Position:** Lay flat on your back with your feet hip-width apart and your knees bent. Arms should be extended by your sides with palms facing down.
2. **Inhale to Prepare:** Take a deep breath in, allowing your abdomen to rise and expand.
3. **Exhale and Lift:** As you exhale, press through your heels and lift your hips towards the ceiling. Engage your glutes and pelvic floor muscles to maintain stability and control.
4. **Hold and Lower:** Hold the bridge position for a few seconds, feeling the activation in your glutes and pelvic floor. After then, gradually return your hips to their initial position.
5. **Repeat:** Focus on keeping the right alignment and control throughout the exercise as you do 10 to 15 repetitions.

TIPS: As you raise your hips off the ground, engage your abdominal muscles and glutes while pressing your heels into the ground.

Rep: 10 to 15

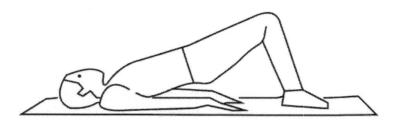

Why You'll Feel the Difference:

Bridge pose targets the glutes, hamstrings, and pelvic floor muscles. By lifting the hips, you engage the glutes while also activating and strengthening the pelvic floor muscles. This exercise helps to improve pelvic stability, enhance core strength, and alleviate tension in the lower back.

LEG SLIDES:

1. **Starting Position:** Lie on your back, bend your knees and place your feet flat on the ground while lying on your back. Your palms should be face downward while you keep your arms at your sides.
2. **Inhale to Prepare:** Take a deep breath in, allowing your abdomen to rise and expand.
3. **Exhale and Slide:** As you exhale, maintain a stable pelvis as you slide one foot away from your body along the floor, keeping the knee bent.
4. **Engage and Return:** Engage your pelvic floor muscles as you gently draw the sliding leg back to the starting position, bringing the knee back in towards your body.
5. **Alternate Sides:** Repeat the movement with the other leg, sliding it away from the body while maintaining pelvic stability and engaging the pelvic floor. Alternate between legs for 10-15 repetitions per side.

REP: ## 10-15 repetitions per side.

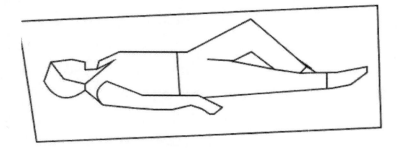

LEG SLIDES

Why You'll Feel the Difference:

Leg slides challenge pelvic stability and control while targeting the hip flexors, inner thighs, and pelvic floor muscles. By maintaining a stable pelvis throughout the movement and engaging the pelvic floor, you strengthen the muscles that support the pelvic organs and improve overall pelvic floor function. This exercise also helps to improve hip mobility and flexibility.

INNER THIGH SQUEEZE:

1. **Starting Position:** Lie on your back, bend your knees and place your feet flat on the ground while lying on your back. Place a small pillow or ball between your knees.
2. **Inhale to Prepare:** Take a deep breath in, allowing your abdomen to rise and expand.
3. **Exhale and Squeeze:** As you exhale, engage your pelvic floor muscles and gently squeeze the pillow or ball between your knees using your inner thigh muscles.
4. **Hold and Release:** Hold the squeeze for a few seconds, feeling the engagement in your inner thighs and pelvic floor. Then, inhale to release the squeeze and allow the pillow or ball to relax.
5. **Repeat:** Perform 10-15 repetitions, focusing on maintaining a steady and controlled squeeze with each repetition.

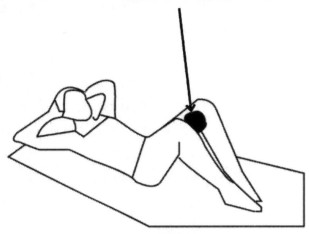

Ball or Pillow

Inner Thigh Squeeze

Why You'll Feel the Difference:

The inner thigh squeeze targets the adductor muscles of the inner thigh and the pelvic floor muscles. By squeezing the pillow or ball, you engage the inner thigh muscles while simultaneously activating the pelvic floor muscles. This exercise helps to strengthen the pelvic floor, improve pelvic stability, and enhance overall lower body strength.

PELVIC CLOCK:

1. **Starting Position:** Lie on your back, bend your knees and place your feet flat on the ground while lying on your back. Keep your hands relaxed at your sides, with the palms facing down.

2. **Imagine the Clock:** Visualize your pelvis as the center of a clock, with 12 o'clock pointing towards your head and 6 o'clock towards your feet.

3. **Tilt Forward:** Inhale to prepare, then exhale as you tilt your pelvis forward towards 12 o'clock, gently arching your lower back away from the floor.

4. **Move to the Right:** Inhale as you tilt your pelvis to the right towards 3 o'clock, feeling a stretch along the left side of your waist.

5. **Tilt Back:** Exhale as you tilt your pelvis back towards 6 o'clock, flattening your lower back against the floor.

6. **Move to the Left:** Inhale as you tilt your pelvis to the left towards 9 o'clock, feeling a stretch along the right side of your waist.
7. **Complete the Circle:** Continue to move your pelvis in a circular motion, clockwise or counterclockwise, making a full circle. Repeat in each direction for five to ten rounds.

Why You'll Feel the Difference:

The pelvic clock exercise helps to improve awareness of pelvic alignment and mobility. By moving the pelvis through different positions, you engage and stretch the muscles surrounding the pelvis, including the pelvic floor muscles. This exercise promotes better pelvic stability, flexibility, and range of motion, which can help alleviate pelvic discomfort and improve overall pelvic health.

SUPINE TOE TAPS:

1. **Starting Position:** Lie on your back, bend your knees and feet flat on the floor. Keep your arms relaxed at your sides, palms down.

2. **Inhale to Prepare:** Take a deep breath in, allowing your abdomen to rise and expand.

3. **Exhale and Extend:** As you exhale, engage your pelvic floor muscles and extend one leg straight out, tapping your toes lightly on the floor while keeping your pelvis stable.

4. **Engage and Return:** Engage your pelvic floor muscles as you bring the extended leg back to the starting position, bending the knee and placing the foot flat on the floor.

5. **Alternate Sides:** Repeat the movement with the other leg, extending it out and tapping the toes while maintaining pelvic stability and engaging the pelvic floor. Alternate between legs for 10-15 repetitions per side.

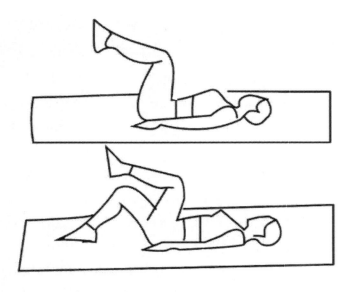

SUPINE TOE TAPS

Why You'll Feel the Difference:

Supine toe taps target the abdominal muscles, hip flexors, and pelvic floor muscles. By extending one leg at a time while keeping the pelvis stable, you challenge pelvic stability and control while also engaging the pelvic floor muscles. This exercise helps to improve pelvic strength, stability, and coordination, which are essential for overall pelvic health and function.

CLAMSHELLS:

1. **Starting Position:** Lie on your side with your knees bent and stacked on top of each other. Rest your head on your bottom arm and keep your hips stacked.

2. **Inhale to Prepare:** Take a deep breath in, allowing your abdomen to rise and expand.

3. **Exhale and Lift:** As you exhale, engage your pelvic floor muscles and lift your top knee towards the ceiling, keeping your feet together. Imagine opening your top knee like a clamshell.

4. **Engage and Lower:** Hold the lifted position for a moment, feeling the engagement in your outer hip and pelvic floor. Then, inhale as you lower your top knee back down with control.

5. **Repeat:** Perform 10-15 repetitions on one side, then switch to the other side and repeat.

Rep: 10-15

Then switch to the other side and repeat.

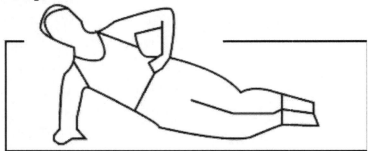

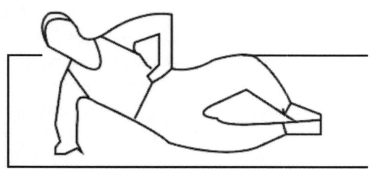

CLAMSHELLS

Why You'll Feel the Difference:

Clamshells target the muscles of the outer hip, including the gluteus medius, while also engaging the pelvic floor muscles. By lifting the knee while keeping the feet together, you activate the muscles responsible for stabilizing the pelvis and improving hip strength and mobility. This exercise helps to prevent hip and pelvic imbalances, improve posture, and alleviate lower back pain.

SEATED HIP OPENER:

1. **Starting Position:** Sit on the edge of a chair with your feet flat on the floor, hip width apart. (You can Place your hands on the sides of the chair for support, keeping your spine tall and shoulders relaxed).
2. **Inhale to Prepare:** Take a deep breath in, allowing your abdomen to rise and expand
3. **Exhale and Open:** As you exhale, engage your pelvic floor muscles and gently open your knees outward, maintaining a comfortable stretch. Keep your feet flat on the floor and avoid any discomfort or strain.
4. **Hold and Release:** Hold the open position for a few seconds, feeling the stretch in your inner thighs and pelvic floor. Then, inhale as you release the tension and bring your knees back together.
5. **Repeat:** Perform 10-15 repetitions, focusing on controlled movement and maintaining proper alignment.

Why You'll Feel the Difference:

Seated hip opener stretches the inner thigh
muscles and promotes flexibility in the hip joints.
Engaging the pelvic floor while opening the
knees, you activate the muscles that support
pelvic stability and alignment. This exercise
helps to improve hip mobility, alleviate tension
in the pelvic area, and enhance overall pelvic
floor function.

PELVIC FLOOR BREATHING:

1. **Starting Position:** Sit comfortably with
   your feet flat on the floor, hip-width apart.
   Place your hands on your thighs or in your
   lap, whichever is comfortable for you.
2. **Inhale Deeply:** Take a slow, deep breath
   in through your nose, allowing your
   abdomen to expand fully. Feel the breath
   filling your belly and pelvis.
3. **Exhale Slowly:** Exhale slowly and gently
   through your mouth, engaging your pelvic
   floor muscles as you exhale. Imagine

gently lifting and drawing in your pelvic floor muscles towards your body.

4. **Repeat:** Continue to inhale deeply through your nose and exhale slowly through your mouth, focusing on engaging your pelvic floor muscles with each exhale. Repeat for 10-15 breaths.

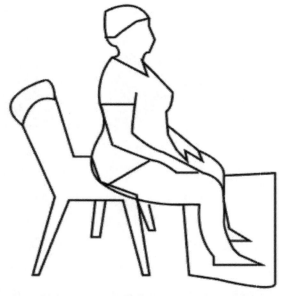

PELVIC FLOOR BREATHING

Why You'll Feel the Difference:

Pelvic floor breathing helps to increase awareness and control of the pelvic floor muscles while promoting relaxation and proper breathing techniques. By consciously engaging the pelvic floor muscles during exhalation, you strengthen and tone the muscles that support pelvic stability and function. This exercise also helps to improve bladder control, alleviate pelvic pain, and enhance overall pelvic floor health.

Chapter 7: Yoga exercises for pelvic floor

Bound Angle Pose (Baddha Konasana):

1. **Starting Position:** Sit on the floor with your legs extended in front of you.
2. **Bring Soles Together:** Bend your knees and bring the soles of your feet together, allowing your knees to fall out to the sides.
3. **Hold Feet:** Hold onto your feet with your hands, interlacing your fingers around your toes.
4. **Sit Tall:** Sit up tall, lengthening through your spine, and engaging your pelvic floor by gently lifting it upwards.
5. **Breathe:** Take deep breaths as you hold the pose, feeling the stretch in your inner thighs and groin area.
6. **Hold:** Hold the pose for 30 seconds to 1 minute, continuing to breathe deeply.

Hold the pose for 30 seconds to 1 minute,

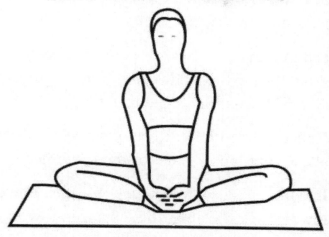

Bound Angle Pose (Baddha Konasana)

Why You'll Feel the Difference:

Bound Angle Pose helps to open up the hips, groin, and inner thighs while also stretching the pelvic floor muscles. By sitting up tall and engaging the pelvic floor, you create stability in the pelvis and support its alignment. This pose can help alleviate tension in the pelvic area, improve flexibility, and promote relaxation.

Child's Pose (Balasana):

Starting Position: Kneel on the floor, sitting back on your heels.

Extend Arms: Lower your forehead to the ground and extend your arms forward or alongside your body, palms facing down.

Relax Pelvic Floor: Relax your pelvic floor and allow your hips to sink towards your heels.

Breathe: Take slow, deep breaths into your lower back, feeling the expansion with each inhale and the release with each exhale.

Hold: Hold the pose for 1-2 minutes, allowing yourself to surrender and relax deeper into the stretch.

Hold the pose for 1-2 minutes

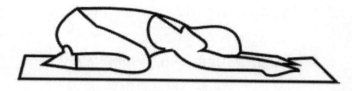

Child's Pose (Balasana)

Why You'll Feel the Difference:

Child's Pose is a gentle resting pose that helps to release tension in the back, shoulders, and hips. When relaxing the pelvic floor and allowing the hips to sink towards the heels, you stretch and release the muscles of the pelvic floor, promoting relaxation and reducing pelvic tension. This pose also helps to calm the mind and relieve stress.

Cat-Cow Stretch:

1. **Starting Position:** Start on your hands and knees in a tabletop position, with your wrists directly under your shoulders and your knees directly under your hips.

2. **Inhale - Cow Pose:** Inhale as you arch your back, dropping your belly towards the floor, lifting your tailbone, and lifting your gaze towards the ceiling.

3. **Exhale - Cat Pose:** As you let your breath out, round your back, tuck your chin into your chest, and pull your belly button toward your spine.

4. **Sync Movement with Breath:** Move between Cow Pose and Cat Pose, flowing with your breath. For the Cat Pose, breathe out, and in for the Cow Pose.

5. **Repeat:** Repeat the sequence for 5-10 rounds, moving slowly and mindfully.

Repeat: 5-10 rounds

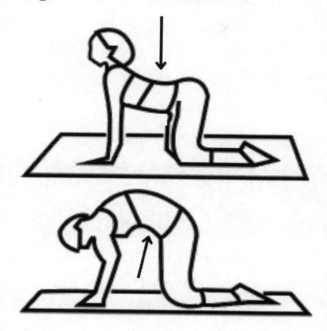

Cat-Cow Stretch

Why You'll Feel the Difference:

The Cat-Cow Stretch helps to improve spinal flexibility and mobility while also gently engaging and stretching the pelvic floor muscles. Moving between the two poses stimulates circulation in the spine, massages the organs in the abdomen, and releases tension in the pelvic area. This dynamic stretch helps to increase awareness of the pelvic floor and can be beneficial for pelvic floor relaxation and strengthening.

Reclining Bound Angle Pose (Supta Baddha Konasana):

1. **Starting Position:** Lie on your back, bend your knees while lying on your back, and feet flat on the floor.
2. **Bring Feet Together:** Allow your knees to fall out to the sides, bringing the soles of your feet together.
3. **Arms Position:** Rest your arms by your sides with palms facing up, allowing your shoulders to relax.
4. **Relax Deeply:** Relax deeply into the pose, allowing gravity to gently open your hips and pelvic floor. You may place cushions

or blocks under your knees for support if needed.

5. **Breathe:** Take slow, deep breaths, allowing your body to surrender and release tension.

6. **Hold:** Hold the pose for 1-2 minutes, continuing to breathe deeply and feeling the gentle opening in your hips and pelvic floor.

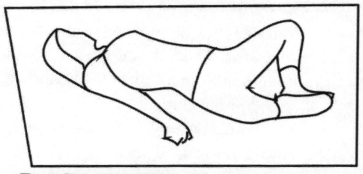

Reclining Bound Angle Pose (Supta Baddha Konasana)

Why You'll Feel the Difference:

Reclining Bound Angle Pose gently opens up the hips and stretches the inner thighs and groin area. If you allow the knees to fall out to the sides and bringing the soles of the feet together, you create a gentle stretch in the pelvic floor muscles. This pose helps to release tension in the hips, improve hip flexibility, and promote relaxation in the pelvic area.

Wide-Legged Forward Fold (Prasarita Padottanasana):

1. **Starting Position:** Stand with your feet wide apart, wider than hip-width distance.
2. **Lengthen Spine:** Inhale to lengthen your spine, lifting through the crown of your head and drawing your shoulders back.
3. **Fold Forward:** Exhale as you hinge at your hips and fold forward, keeping your spine long and your chest open. Bring your hands to the floor or onto blocks for support.
4. **Relax Head:** Allow your head to relax towards the floor, releasing any tension in your neck and shoulders.

5. **Feel the Stretch:** Feel a gentle stretch in your inner thighs and pelvic floor as you fold forward.

6. **Breathe:** Take slow, deep breaths, allowing your body to relax deeper into the stretch.

7. **Hold:** Hold the pose for 30 seconds to 1 minute, continuing to breathe deeply and feeling the stretch in your pelvic area.

Hold: 30 seconds to 1 minute

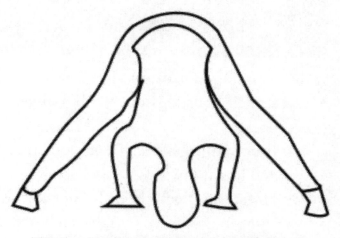

Wide-Legged Forward Fold (Prasarita Padottanasana)

Why You'll Feel the Difference:

Wide-Legged Forward Fold stretches the inner thighs, hamstrings, and pelvic floor muscles. When you fold forward with wide legs, you create space and length in the pelvic area, promoting flexibility and mobility. This pose helps to release tension in the pelvic floor, improve circulation, and calm the mind.

Reclining Hand-to-Big-Toe Pose (Supta Padangusthasana):

1. **Starting Position:** Lie on your back, stretch your legs out while lying on your back.
2. **Bend Right Knee:** Bend your right knee and hug it towards your chest.
3. **Hold Big Toe:** Hold the big toe of your right foot with your right hand, extending your left hand out to the side for balance.
4. **Extend Right Leg:** Extend your right leg towards the ceiling, keeping it straight and engaged.

5. **Feel the Stretch:** Feel a stretch along the back of your right leg, targeting the hamstrings and calf muscles.
6. **Breathe:** Take slow, deep breaths, allowing your body to relax into the stretch.
7. **Hold:** Hold the pose for 30 seconds to 1 minute, continuing to breathe deeply and feeling the stretch in your right leg.
8. **Switch Sides:** Release your right leg and repeat the pose on the left side.

- ## Hold: 30 seconds to 1 minute
- ## Switch Sides

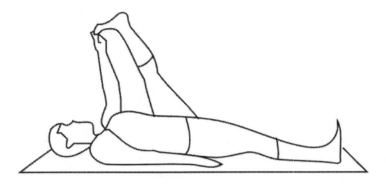

Reclining Hand-to-Big-Toe Pose
(Supta Padangusthasana)

Why You'll Feel the Difference:

Reclining Hand-to-Big-Toe Pose stretches the hamstrings, calves, and pelvic floor muscles. By extending the leg towards the ceiling, you create a deep stretch along the back of the leg and into the pelvic area. This pose helps to improve flexibility in the hamstrings, relieve tension in the pelvic floor, and promote relaxation.

Happy Baby Pose (Ananda Balasana):

1. **Starting Position:** Lie on your back, bend your knees while lying down and feet flat on the floor.
2. **Draw Knees Towards Chest:** Bring your knees towards your chest, keeping them bent.
3. **Hold Feet:** Reach for the outside edges of your feet with your hands, grabbing onto your toes or ankles.
4. **Bring Knees to Armpits:** Gently bring your knees towards your armpits, allowing your thighs to come closer to your torso.
5. **Rock Side to Side:** Rock gently from side to side, massaging your lower back and pelvic floor.
6. **Hold:** Hold the pose for 30 seconds to 1 minute, breathing deeply and relaxing into the stretch.

- **Hold: 30 seconds to 1 minute**
- **Breathing deeply and relaxing into the stretch**

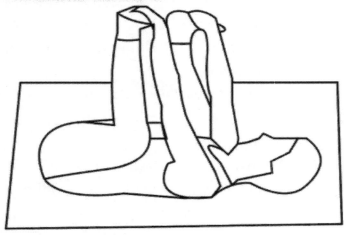

Happy Baby Pose (Ananda Balasana)

Why You'll Feel the Difference:

Happy Baby Pose helps to stretch the inner thighs, groin, and lower back while also releasing tension in the pelvic floor muscles. By drawing the knees towards the armpits and holding onto the feet, you create a deep stretch in the pelvic area. This pose promotes relaxation, relieves lower back pain, and improves hip flexibility.

Supine Twist (Supta Matsyendrasana):

1. **Starting Position:** Lie on your back with your arms extended out to the sides in a T position.
2. **Lift Feet Off Floor:** Bend your knees and lift your feet off the floor, bringing your shins parallel to the floor.
3. **Lower Knees:** Exhale as you lower your knees to one side, keeping both shoulders grounded on the floor.
4. **Hold:** Hold the twist for 30 seconds to 1 minute, allowing your spine to gently rotate and release tension.
5. **Switch Sides:** Inhale as you lift your knees back to center, then exhale as you lower them to the opposite side. The other side should be held for the same amount of time.

- **Hold: 30 seconds to 1 minute**
- **Switch Sides**

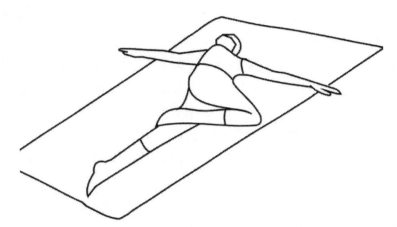

Supine Twist (Supta Matsyendrasana)

Why You'll Feel the Difference:

Supine Twist stretches the spine, shoulders, and chest while also providing a gentle massage to the abdominal organs and pelvic floor muscles. Twisting the spine, you release tension and improve spinal mobility, which can alleviate back pain and improve posture. This pose also aids in digestion and detoxification.

Legs-Up-The-Wall Pose (Viparita Karani):

1. **Starting Position:** Sit close to a wall with your side facing the wall.
2. **Lie Back:** Lie on your back and extend your legs up the wall, allowing your heels to rest against the wall.
3. **Arms Position:** Keep your arms by your sides with palms facing up, allowing your shoulders to relax.
4. **Relax Deeply:** Relax deeply into the pose, allowing gravity to gently stretch your pelvic floor and lower back.
5. **Hold:** Hold the pose for 5-10 minutes, focusing on deep, relaxed breathing and allowing your body to release tension.

- ## Hold the pose for 5-10 minutes

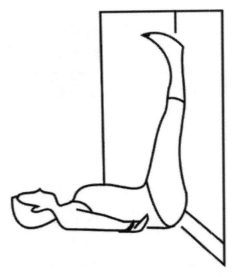

Legs-Up-The-Wall Pose (Viparita Karani)

Why You'll Feel the Difference:

Legs-Up-The-Wall Pose is a restorative pose that promotes relaxation and relieves tension in the lower body, including the pelvic floor muscles. Elevating the legs above the heart, you improve circulation and reduce swelling in the legs and feet. This pose also helps to calm the nervous system, reduce stress, and promote better sleep.

Supported Bridge Pose:

1. **Starting Position:** Lie on your back, bend your knees while lying down and feet flat on the floor, hip-width apart.
2. **Prepare the Support:** Place a yoga block or bolster under your sacrum, the triangular bone at the base of your spine, ensuring it's positioned comfortably and securely.
3. **Adjustment:** You may need to adjust the height of the block or bolster to find the most supportive position for your body.
4. **Press into Feet:** Press firmly into your feet, activating your leg muscles.
5. **Lift Hips:** On an exhale, slowly lift your hips towards the ceiling, engaging your glutes and pelvic floor muscles. Keep your spine in a neutral position without overarching your lower back.

6. **Support Arms:** Relax your arms by your sides, palms facing down, or interlace your fingers underneath you, rolling your shoulders underneath you to open the chest.
7. **Hold:** Hold the pose for 30 seconds to 1 minute, maintaining steady breathing and focusing on engaging your glutes and pelvic floor muscles.
8. **Release:** To release the pose, gently lower your hips back down to the floor and remove the support from underneath you.

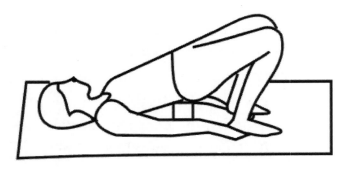

Supported Bridge Pose

Why You'll Feel the Difference:

Supported Bridge Pose opens up the chest, shoulders, and hip flexors while also strengthening the glutes and engaging the pelvic floor muscles. By elevating the hips on a block or bolster, you create space in the lower back and pelvis, relieving tension and compression in the spine. This pose helps to improve posture, alleviate lower back pain, and promote relaxation. Also, engaging the pelvic floor muscles in this pose helps to strengthen and tone them, contributing to better pelvic health and stability.

Bonus Section:

Common Myths and Misconceptions About Pelvic Floor Exercises

Pelvic floor exercises, also known as Kegel exercises, have gained significant attention in recent years due to their numerous benefits in promoting pelvic health and addressing issues such as urinary incontinence, pelvic organ prolapse, and sexual dysfunction. However, along with this increased awareness, several myths and misconceptions have emerged. Here, we'll address common myths and misconceptions about pelvic floor exercises:

Myth: Pelvic floor exercises are only for women.

Fact: Both men and women have pelvic floor muscles, and pelvic floor exercises are beneficial for both genders. Men can also experience urinary incontinence and pelvic floor dysfunction, making these exercises equally important for them.

Myth: Pelvic floor exercises are only for older adults.

Fact: Pelvic floor exercises are beneficial for individuals of all ages, including young adults and even children. Strengthening these muscles early in life can help prevent pelvic floor issues later on.

Myth: Pelvic floor exercises are only for individuals who have pelvic floor dysfunction.

Fact: Pelvic floor exercises can benefit everyone, regardless of whether they have pelvic floor issues. Strengthening these muscles can improve bladder and bowel control, enhance sexual function, and support overall pelvic health.

Myth: Pelvic floor exercises are the same as doing squats or keg stands.

Fact: While squats and certain yoga poses may engage the pelvic floor muscles to some extent, they are not targeted pelvic floor exercises like Kegels. The muscles on the floor of the pelvis are worked out especially by Kegel movements.

Myth: Pelvic floor exercises are difficult and time-consuming.

Fact: Pelvic floor exercises can be simple and quick to perform. They can be done discreetly anywhere, anytime, making them easy to incorporate into daily routines.

Myth: You'll see immediate results from pelvic floor exercises.

Fact: Like any muscle-strengthening regimen, results from pelvic floor exercises may take time to become noticeable. Consistency is key, and it may take weeks or months to see significant improvements.

Myth: Pelvic floor exercises are only for individuals who have given birth.

Fact: While childbirth can weaken the pelvic floor muscles, anyone can benefit from pelvic floor exercises, regardless of whether they've given birth or not.

Myth: Pelvic floor exercises are only for individuals with urinary incontinence.

Fact: While pelvic floor exercises are often recommended for urinary incontinence, they also help with other pelvic floor issues such as pelvic organ prolapse, fecal incontinence, and sexual dysfunction.

Myth: You only need to do pelvic floor exercises when you have symptoms.

Fact: Pelvic floor exercises are beneficial for prevention as well as treatment. Strengthening these muscles can help prevent pelvic floor issues from developing or worsening over time.

Myth: Pelvic floor exercises are only effective for mild cases of urinary incontinence.

Fact: Pelvic floor exercises can be effective for various degrees of urinary incontinence, including mild, moderate, and even severe cases. They may also be used as part of a comprehensive treatment plan alongside other interventions.

Myth: Pelvic floor exercises are unnecessary if you've had surgery for pelvic organ prolapse.

Fact: Pelvic floor exercises are often recommended as part of the post-surgery recovery process for pelvic organ prolapse. Strengthening the pelvic floor muscles can help support the surgical repair and reduce the risk of recurrence.

Myth: You don't need to do pelvic floor exercises if you've had a cesarean section.

Fact: Pregnancy itself can weaken the pelvic floor muscles, regardless of the delivery method. Pelvic floor exercises are beneficial for all pregnant individuals, including those who have had a cesarean section.

Myth: Pelvic floor exercises are only for individuals with bladder issues.

Fact: While pelvic floor exercises are often associated with bladder control, they also play a crucial role in bowel function, sexual function, and overall pelvic health.

Myth: You'll develop stronger pelvic floor muscles by doing more repetitions of Kegels.

Fact: Like any muscle group, the pelvic floor muscles require a balance of strength and endurance. Doing too many repetitions of Kegels without proper rest can lead to muscle fatigue and overexertion.

Myth: Pelvic floor exercises are only for individuals who are sexually active.

Fact: Pelvic floor exercises are beneficial for everyone, regardless of their sexual activity status. Strengthening these muscles can improve bladder and bowel control, support pelvic organ health, and enhance overall quality of life.

Myth: Pelvic floor exercises are ineffective for men with erectile dysfunction.

Fact: Pelvic floor exercises, particularly those that target the bulbocavernosus muscle, can improve erectile function in men by enhancing blood flow to the penis and promoting better control over ejaculation.

Myth: Pelvic floor exercises are only for individuals with weakened pelvic floor muscles.

Fact: Pelvic floor exercises can benefit individuals with both weak and tight pelvic floor muscles. For those with tight pelvic floor muscles, relaxation techniques may be more appropriate.

Myth: You only need to do pelvic floor exercises during pregnancy.

Fact: While pelvic floor exercises are important during pregnancy to support the added weight of the uterus, they are beneficial for pelvic health throughout life. Regular exercise can help prevent pelvic floor issues from developing later on.

Myth: Pelvic floor exercises can't help with chronic pelvic pain.

Fact: Pelvic floor exercises, along with other interventions such as physical therapy and relaxation techniques, can help alleviate symptoms of chronic pelvic pain by improving muscle function and reducing tension in the pelvic floor muscles.

Myth: You don't need to do pelvic floor exercises if you're not experiencing any symptoms.

Fact: Pelvic floor exercises are beneficial for everyone, regardless of whether they have symptoms of pelvic floor dysfunction. Strengthening these muscles can help prevent issues from arising in the future and support overall pelvic health and function.

Frequently asked questions and answer

What are pelvic floor muscle exercises?

Pelvic floor muscle exercises, also known as Kegel exercises, are a series of exercises designed to strengthen and tone the muscles of the pelvic floor.

Why are pelvic floor muscle exercises important for senior women?

Pelvic floor muscle exercises are important for senior women to maintain bladder and bowel control, support pelvic organ health, improve sexual function, and prevent pelvic floor issues such as urinary incontinence and pelvic organ prolapse.

How do I know if I need to do pelvic floor muscle exercises?

If you experience symptoms such as urinary leakage, frequent urination, difficulty controlling bowel movements, pelvic pressure or discomfort, or sexual dysfunction, pelvic floor muscle exercises may be beneficial.

Can pelvic floor muscle exercises help with urinary incontinence?

Yes, pelvic floor muscle exercises are often recommended as a first-line treatment for urinary incontinence. Strengthening these muscles can improve bladder control and reduce episodes of leakage.

How do I perform pelvic floor muscle exercises?

To perform pelvic floor muscle exercises, contract the muscles of your pelvic floor as if you're trying to stop the flow of urine. Hold for a few seconds, then relax. Repeat for multiple repetitions, gradually increasing the duration of each contraction.

How often should I do pelvic floor muscle exercises?

Aim to do pelvic floor muscle exercises at least three times per day. Start with a small number of repetitions and gradually increase over time as your muscles become stronger.

Can I do pelvic floor muscle exercises if I have pelvic organ prolapse?

Yes, pelvic floor muscle exercises can be beneficial for individuals with pelvic organ prolapse. However, it's essential to work with a healthcare professional to ensure you're performing the exercises correctly and to determine the appropriate intensity for your condition.

Are there any risks associated with pelvic floor muscle exercises?

Pelvic floor muscle exercises are generally safe for most individuals. However, performing the exercises incorrectly or overexerting the muscles can lead to muscle strain or exacerbate existing pelvic floor issues. It's essential to learn proper technique and listen to your body's signals.

Can I do pelvic floor muscle exercises during pregnancy?

Yes, pelvic floor muscle exercises are safe and beneficial during pregnancy to support the added weight of the uterus and prevent issues such as urinary incontinence and pelvic organ prolapse. For specific advice, it is essential to speak with a healthcare provider, nevertheless.

Can pelvic floor muscle exercises improve sexual function in senior women?

Yes, pelvic floor muscle exercises can improve sexual function in senior women by increasing pelvic blood flow, enhancing vaginal tone, and improving sensation and arousal.

How long does it take to see results from pelvic floor muscle exercises?

The time it takes to see results from pelvic floor muscle exercises varies from person to person. Some individuals may notice improvements in bladder control within a few weeks, while others may take longer. Consistency is key.

Are there any specific pelvic floor muscle exercises for senior women?

While the basic technique of pelvic floor muscle exercises is the same for everyone, there are variations and modifications that may be more suitable for senior women, such as exercises performed in a seated or lying position.

Can I do pelvic floor muscle exercises if I have osteoporosis?

Yes, pelvic floor muscle exercises are generally safe for individuals with osteoporosis. However, it's essential to avoid high-impact exercises that may put excessive strain on the bones. Low-impact exercises such as Kegels are recommended.

Can pelvic floor muscle exercises help with pelvic pain?

Yes, pelvic floor muscle exercises can help alleviate pelvic pain by improving muscle function, reducing muscle tension, and promoting relaxation in the pelvic floor muscles.

How do I know if I'm performing pelvic floor muscle exercises correctly?

To ensure you're performing pelvic floor muscle exercises correctly, focus on isolating the pelvic floor muscles without contracting the buttocks, abdomen, or thighs. You should feel a tightening and lifting sensation in the pelvic area.

Can I do pelvic floor muscle exercises if I've had pelvic surgery?

In many cases, pelvic floor muscle exercises are beneficial for individuals who have had pelvic surgery. However, it's essential to consult with your healthcare provider to ensure the exercises are safe and appropriate for your specific situation.

Can I do pelvic floor muscle exercises if I have a prolapsed bladder or uterus?

Yes, pelvic floor muscle exercises can help strengthen the muscles that support the bladder and uterus, potentially reducing symptoms of prolapse. However, it's essential to work with a healthcare professional to determine the appropriate exercises and intensity for your condition.

Can I do pelvic floor muscle exercises if I'm not sure if I'm doing them correctly?

If you're unsure whether you're performing pelvic floor muscle exercises correctly, consider seeking guidance from a pelvic floor physical therapist or healthcare provider. They can assess your technique and provide personalized recommendations.

Are there any devices or tools that can help with pelvic floor muscle exercises?

Yes, there are various devices available, such as vaginal weights or biofeedback devices, that can help enhance pelvic floor muscle exercises by providing feedback or resistance. However, these tools are not necessary for everyone and should be used under the guidance of a healthcare professional.

Can I do pelvic floor muscle exercises if I have arthritis?

Yes, pelvic floor muscle exercises are generally safe for individuals with arthritis. However, it's essential to choose exercises and modifications that are comfortable for your joints and to avoid any movements that cause pain or discomfort.

Can I do pelvic floor muscle exercises if I have mobility limitations?

Yes, pelvic floor muscle exercises can be adapted to accommodate individuals with mobility limitations. Exercises can be performed in a seated or lying position, and modifications can be made as needed to ensure safety and comfort.

Are there any dietary or lifestyle changes that can complement pelvic floor muscle exercises?

Yes, maintaining a healthy lifestyle, including staying hydrated, maintaining a healthy weight, and avoiding constipation, can complement pelvic floor muscle exercises and promote overall pelvic health.

Can I do pelvic floor muscle exercises if I'm undergoing treatment for cancer?

In many cases, pelvic floor muscle exercises are safe for individuals undergoing cancer treatment. However, it's essential to consult with your healthcare provider to ensure the exercises are appropriate for your specific situation and treatment plan.

Can I do pelvic floor muscle exercises if I have a history of pelvic trauma or abuse?

Individuals with a history of pelvic trauma or abuse may find pelvic floor muscle exercises challenging or triggering.

Can I stop doing pelvic floor muscle exercises once I see improvement in my symptoms?

Pelvic floor muscle exercises are most effective when performed consistently as part of a long-term pelvic health maintenance plan. Once symptoms improve, it's essential to continue with a maintenance routine to prevent issues from recurring.

Conclusion

In conclusion, pelvic floor muscle exercises are a valuable tool for senior women to maintain pelvic health, prevent pelvic floor issues, and enhance overall quality of life. By addressing frequently asked questions and dispelling common misconceptions, you can better understand the importance of pelvic floor exercises and how to incorporate them into their daily routine.

Through regular practice of pelvic floor muscle exercises, senior women can strengthen the muscles that support the bladder, bowel, and uterus, thereby improving bladder and bowel control, reducing symptoms of urinary incontinence and pelvic organ prolapse, and enhancing sexual function. These exercises also promote pelvic floor relaxation, alleviate pelvic pain, and support overall pelvic health and well-being.

Incorporating pelvic floor muscle exercises into your daily routine doesn't have to be complicated or time-consuming. With consistency and dedication, you can gradually strengthen your pelvic floor muscles and experience improvements in bladder and bowel function, pelvic support, and overall quality of life.

Whether you're experiencing pelvic floor issues or simply looking to maintain pelvic health as you age, pelvic floor muscle exercises are a valuable tool that can support you on your journey to optimal health and wellness.

Appreciation and Encouragement

To all those who have taken the time to read this book and look into the world of pelvic floor muscle exercises, I extend my heartfelt appreciation and admiration. Your commitment to learning and understanding your pelvic health is commendable, and I applaud your dedication to taking proactive steps towards improving your well-being.

*Embarking on a journey to better pelvic health requires **courage, persistence, and a willingness** to embrace change. By engaging with the information presented in this book, you have demonstrated a genuine desire to prioritize your health and empower yourself with knowledge and tools to promote pelvic wellness.*

*I encourage you to approach your pelvic floor exercises with **enthusiasm and determination**. Remember that every repetition, every contraction, and every moment of mindful engagement with your pelvic floor muscles brings you one step closer to achieving your health goals.*

While the road to pelvic health may have its challenges, I want to reassure you that you are not alone on this journey. There is a vast community of individuals, healthcare professionals, and resources available to support you every step of the way.

*As you embark on this path, I urge you to be **patient and compassionate** with yourself. Rome wasn't built in a day, and neither is pelvic health achieved overnight. Celebrate your progress, no matter how small, and recognize that every effort you make towards strengthening your pelvic floor muscles is a significant investment in your overall well-being.*

***Lastly,** I want to remind you that your health journey is unique to you. Trust in your instincts, listen to your body, and honor your needs along the way. You have the power to shape your health and create a future filled with vitality, strength, and resilience.*

*So, keep moving forward with confidence, determination, and a sense of purpose. Your pelvic health journey is worth every step, and I believe in your ability to achieve your goals and thrive. **You've got this!***

Made in the USA
Columbia, SC
16 May 2024

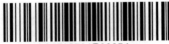

35709701R00054